HOW TO MAKE HAND SANITIZER GEL

THE EASY GUIDE TO MAKING YOUR HAND SANITIZER AT HOME

© **Copyright 2020-All rights Reserved!**

This record prepared towards giving exact and reliable information concerning the subject and issue made sure about. The dispersion sold with the likelihood that the wholesaler isn't required to render accounting, definitively permitted, or something different, qualified organizations.

The information gave right now, to be completely forthright and consistent, in that any commitment, concerning absentmindedness or something different, by any use or abuse of any courses of action, methodology, or headings contained inside is the sole and eloquent obligation of the recipient examines. In no way, form will any lawful commitment or deficiency be held against the merchant for any reparation, hurts, or monetary disaster due to the information; along these lines, either direct or in an indirect way.

TABLE OF CONTENTS

Introduction —————————————————————————— 6

    GUIDELINES OF HAND SANITIZERS BY FDA ——————— 8

    What Are the Benefits of Using Hand Sanitizer? ——————— 9

RECIPES OF HAND SANITIZERS ————————————————— 11

    Step by step instructions to make your hand sanitizer: List of fixings ———————————————————————————— 11

        1st Recipe ————————————————————————— 11

        2nd Recipe ———————————————————————— 12

        3rd Recipe ————————————————————————— 12

        4th Recipe ————————————————————————— 13

        5th Recipe ————————————————————————— 14

        Alternative Recipe ———————————————————— 14

        6th Recipe ————————————————————————— 15

When to use Hand sanitizer ————————————————————— 17

    The most effective method to utilize hand sanitizer ——————— 17

    Why is proper cleaning necessary for hands? ————————— 18

Hand Washing with Sanitizer and Water ———————————————— 20

    Would it be good for me to use Hand sanitizer? ——————— 20

    What type of hand sanitizer should you use? ———————— 21

    How to use Hand sanitizer? ———————————————— 21

When Does hand sanitizer does not work? ---------------------- 21

WHERE DO BACTERIAL INFECTIONS GENERATE ------------- 24

Decreased Susceptibility of Bacteria to Cleaning agents ----------- 24

Critical Locations for Hand Sanitizer --------------------------- 25

Exchange counters -- 27

Choosing the Right-Hand Sanitizer --------------------------- 27

Empowering Hand Hygiene --------------------------------------- 28

Sterilizing the Workplace -- 28

CONCLUSION --- 29

DESCRIPTION

Hand sanitizer is become necessary to fight for the germs, viruses and bacterial infections we are dealing with now a days by understanding the need of todays world health condition I decided to write a book for the people who want there family friends and themselves to be on safe side. By knowing the lacking of sanitizer in your era we decided to teach you how to make your own hand sanitizer without spending too much, I hope it will help you in your daily life and keep you safe and sound

CHAPTER 1
INTRODUCTION

Hand Sanitizer is broadly utilized on the planet when there is a constrained wellspring of cleanser and water (Franklin 2006). In the wake of using the latrine, and before planning or eating nourishment, it is essential to wash your hands or use hand sanitizer, and many picks with the following option (Wonderly 2011). Most hand sanitizers have ethyl liquor as a principle fixing, while others that don't have it, as a rule, use triclosan to eliminate microscopic organisms. It realized that alcohol-based hand sanitizers are more compelling than non-liquor ones. Since liquor based hand sanitizers most broadly used, Purell, an alcohol-based hand sanitizer, was tried in the examination.

Numerous individuals on the planet depend close by sanitizer for everyday use, and it is significant for these individuals to realize whether hand sanitizer is viable enough (Franklin 2006). Purell was consistently tried in labs and not in ordinary home utilization. Along these, the reason for this investigation is to decide if Purell is viable in eliminating microbes. By testing the effectivity of Purell, we will have a superior comprehension of what they ought to use to sterilize their hands (Sohn 2013).

Liquid hand sanitizers - for the most part, liquor based gels - have delighted in a blast in notoriety over the most recent ten years. If you have gone via plane or gone to a study hall in the U.S. of late, odds are you have seen hand sanitizers used.

Hand sanitizers don't fill in as a swap for careful handwashing. Instead, they thought to bring purchasers a portion of the advantages of handwashing when handwashing isn't functional.

The adequacy of hand sanitizer relies upon various elements, remembering the way for which the item applied (e.g., amount utilized, length of introduction, recurrence of utilization) and whether the particular irresistible specialists present on the individual's hands are vulnerable to the dynamic fixing in the product.

as a rule, liquor based hand sanitizers, altogether over finger and hand surfaces for a time of 30 seconds, trailed by complete air-drying, can successfully decrease populaces of microorganisms, organisms, and some encompassed infections (e.g., flu A viruses).1,6,9 Similar impacts have been accounted for specific liquor-free details, for example, SAB (surfactant, allantoin, and BAC) hand sanitizer.1,3,8 Most hand sanitizers, notwithstanding, are moderately ineffectual against bacterial spores, nonenveloped infections (e.g., norovirus), and encysted parasites (e.g., Giardia). They additionally don't wholly wash down or disinfect the skin when hands are recognizably dirty preceding application.

Epidemiological examinations have not solidly settled the connection between hand sanitizer use and decreased ailment. Yet, a few research centre investigations recommend hand sanitizers help to forestall diseases by executing transient pathogenic microscopic organisms.

Handwashing and hand sanitizers diminish microbial populaces in various manners. Handwashing - regardless of whether finished with "antibacterial" cleanser or everyday cleanser - indeed expels microorganisms from the skin, actually washing the live organisms down the channel. Hand sanitizers diminish levels of microorganisms by executing them artificially, much the same as disinfectants eliminate germs on natural surfaces.

The extent of the impact of handwashing is, for the most part, and the element of wash time and cleanser utilization. Washing hands without cleanser are significantly less powerful. Viability from hand sanitizers is best when an enormous volume of item applied to the sides. Using a massive quantity of hand sanitizer guarantees overabundance dynamic fixing and expands the time of synthetic movement before the hand sanitizer dissipates.

In contrast to disinfectants, which might be left for all intents and purposes on surfaces for up to around 5 minutes, hand sanitizers must carry out their responsibility inside a short timeframe to create the fundamental impact. A great many people just won't endure wet hands for more than around 30 seconds. In like manner, Microchem

Laboratory accepts that 30 seconds - possibly one moment in uncommon cases - ought to be the contact time limit for lab testing of hand sanitizers.

Various distinctive dynamic fixings might fuel hand sanitizers; however, have you at any point seen that most hand sanitizers use liquor as the dynamic fixing? That is generally an aftereffect of how they controlled.

GUIDELINES OF HAND SANITIZERS BY FDA

Hand sanitizers are directed in the USA by the Food and Drug Administration (FDA) as medications. In 1994, the FDA distributed a record called the "Conditional Final Monograph for OTC Healthcare Antiseptic Drug Products." It is regularly referred to in the business as the TFM. The album, however "conditional," fills in as a guide to testing prerequisites and covers a wide range of antimicrobials intended to apply to the skin, including hand sanitizers. FDA is keen on settling the monograph; however, it isn't relied upon to be finished at any point soon.

Organizations keen on promoting a hand sanitizer in the United States will profit by getting comfortable with the FDA Tentative Final Monograph. Areas of the FDA Tentative Final Monograph follow, with portions highlighted and talked about in further detail. Keep in mind, the tables and segments talked about underneath originate from the conditional last monograph, so there's space to alter and streamline reads for accommodation to administrative organizations.

Notwithstanding the fluctuation in viability, hand sanitizers can help control the transmission of irresistible ailments, particularly in settings where consistency with handwashing is weak. For instance, among kids in grade schools, the joining of either a liquor based or an alcohol-free hand sanitizer into study hall hand-cleanliness programs has been related with decreases in truancy identified with irresistible illness.10,11 Likewise, in the work environment, the utilization of liquor based hand sanitizer has been associated with reductions in disease scenes and debilitated days.12 In emergency clinics and human services facilities, expanded access to alcohol-based hand sanitizer has been connected to by and significant enhancements close by the cleanliness

Offices, for example, the World Health Organization and the U.S. Communities for Disease Control and Prevention advance the utilization of liquor based hand sanitizers over liquor-free products.2,15,16 Indeed, the use of liquor-free items has stayed restricted, to a limited extent on account of WHO's and CDC's attention on liquor based items yet also in light of worries about the wellbeing of synthetics utilized in liquor-free items. Research has shown that specific antimicrobial mixes, for example, triclosan, for instance, may meddle with the capacity of the endocrine system.17 Environmental pollution from triclosan is another concern.18 Disinfectants and antimicrobials additionally can conceivably add to the advancement of antimicrobial resistance.1,7,15 In 2014, mounting worries over triclosan drove experts in the European Union (E.U.) to limit the substance's utilization in different shopper items in the E.U.

By correlation, worries over the utilization of liquor based hand sanitizer have focused fundamentally on item combustibility and ingestion, both inadvertent (e.g., by small kids) and deliberate (by people looking to manhandle alcohol).6,20,21 With appropriate capacity and techniques that limit access to liquor containing sanitizer (e.g., giving hand sanitizer to people), the danger of fire or harming from incidental or purposeful ingestion of alcohol based hand sanitizers viewed as low

WHAT ARE THE BENEFITS OF USING HAND SANITIZER?

Liquor based sanitizers help to prevent the spread of germs and ailment causing microorganisms, especially in occupied situations like schools, parks and workplaces:

According to examines, 1 of every five individuals don't frequently wash hands. Of the individuals who do, 70% don't utilize cleanser. Giving hand sanitizer in critical zones (counting restrooms and kitchens) makes it more probable that individuals will use it to slaughter destructive microorganisms.

Advance Good Hygiene and Health: A sound structure is a gainful one. One examination in the American Journal of Infection Control (AJIC) found that empowering the utilization of hand sanitizers in schools decreased non-appearance by practically 20%!

Decrease Waste: As an additional safety measure, numerous individuals will utilize paper towels to open entryways when leaving restrooms or kitchens. Putting hand sanitizers close to exits makes it simple for individuals to shield themselves from germs without expecting to make extra chaos.

Do you know the tips and deceives for successful handwashing? Look at this infographic to review your insight!

CHAPTER 2

RECIPES OF HAND SANITIZERS

There are several recipes which used to make homemade sanitizers but for your help and well being we have collected some methods which are easy to make and will benefit you and your loved ones

STEP BY STEP INSTRUCTIONS TO MAKE YOUR HAND SANITIZER: LIST OF FIXINGS

A hand sanitizer comprises of a fundamental equation, and it's anything but difficult to make your own at home if your neighbourhood drug store or retailer is coming up short. These are the fixings you'll require:

1ST RECIPE

- 2/3 cup 99.9% isopropyl liquor. You can discover isopropyl liquor at any drugstore or drug store if it's out of stock at Amazon. A one-quart container ought to be accessible for around $15, and you'll have the option to make a great deal of hand sanitizer with that. On the off chance that you like being erring on the side of caution, you can likewise get a six-quart pack.
- 1/3 cup 98% aloe vera gel. You have to blend the isopropyl liquor with something because on its own it will consume your hands. The perfect arrangement is aloe vera gel as it goes about as a characteristic cream.
- 8 - 10 drops of fundamental oils. If you have to add some aroma to the blend, get a pack of essential oils. It isn't required. However, most pocket hand sanitizers nowadays have some perfume, and in case you're utilized to the smell, it doesn't cost a lot to get a couple of essential oils.
- Bowl and spoon to combine everything.

- An essential pipe to get your hand sanitizer into a container.
- Plastic travel bottles for putting away the hand sanitizer. When you prepare your hand sanitizer, you'll need containers to convey it in. You can get a six-pack of 2oz containers for $7, and they accompany a flip top that makes it simple to press out the hand sanitizer. In case you're making hand sanitizer for home use, you can get a six-pack of 8oz containers for just $9.
- Nitrile gloves so you don't consume your hands when making the hand sanitizer

2ND RECIPE

- Isopropyl liquor
- Aloe vera gel
- Tea tree oil

Blend 3 sections isopropyl liquor to 1 section aloe vera gel. Include drops of tea tree oil to give it a pleasant fragrance and to adjust your chakras.

3RD RECIPE

- Isopropyl liquor
- Glycerol
- Hydrogen peroxide
- Refined water
- Shower bottle

1. The aloe blend takes care of business. However, aloe additionally leaves your skin annoyingly clingy. Along these lines, here's a formula that is not so much clingy but slightly more intense, in light of the blend prescribed by the WHO.
2. Blend 1 ⅔ cups liquor with two teaspoons of glycerol. You can purchase containers of glycerol on the web, and it's a significant fixing since it shields the alcohol from drying out your hands. On the off chance that you can't discover glycerol, continue

with the remainder of the formula at any rate and simply make sure to saturate your hands in the wake of applying the sanitizer.

3. Blend in 1 tablespoon of hydrogen peroxide, at that point another ¼ cup of refined or bubbled (at that point cooled) water. (In case you're working with a lower-fixation arrangement of scouring liquor, use far less water; recall, in any event, ⅔ of your last blend must be liquor.)
4. Burden the arrangement into shower bottles—this isn't a gel, it's a splash. You can wet a paper towel also and utilize that as a wipe.
5. If you should, you can include a sprinkle of organic oil to your invention to make it smell pleasant. Simply don't utilize lavender. Every other person uses lavender, and your sanitizer is unrivalled.

4TH RECIPE

- Two sections isopropyl Liquor or ethanol (91 per cent to 99 per cent liquor)
- one section aloe vera
- A couple of drops of clove, eucalyptus, peppermint, or other fundamental oil.
- On the off chance that you are making hand sanitizer at home, Khubchandani says to cling to these tips:
- Make the hand sanitizer in a perfect space. Wipe down ledges with a weakened fade arrangement in advance.
- Wash your hands before making the hand sanitizer.
- To blend, utilize a perfect spoon and whisk. Wash these things altogether before using them.
- Ensure the liquor utilized for the hand sanitizer weakened.

Blend all the fixings altogether until they are all around mixed.] Try not to contact the blend with your hands until it prepared for use.

5TH RECIPE

For a bigger group of hand sanitizer, the World Health Organization (WHO)Trusted Source has a recipe for a hand sanitizer that employments:

- isopropyl Liquor or ethanol
- Hydrogen peroxide
- glycerol
- sterile refined or bubbled cold water
- Hand Sanitizer

For those occasions when past cleanser and water simply aren't accessible, and hands should wash, keep a custom made hand sanitizer (made with a couple of fundamental fixings) in your sack.

ALTERNATIVE RECIPE

- 3 TB 190 proof liquor or if nothing else 120 proof or scouring liquor or witch hazel (the first formula called witch hazel, nonetheless, alcohol is viewed as the best)
- 1 T.B. aloe vera (this is to keep hands from drying out from the liquor)
- 1/2 tsp vegetable glycerin or nutrient E oil
- 20 drops tea tree fundamental oil
- 10 drops lavender fundamental oil

DIRECTIONS

Consolidate all the fixings in a bowl. To utilize the hand sanitizer store in a little container or a press tube (this way). This formula will make two liquid ounces (one cylinder.) If you like to take a shower, utilize this formula.

6TH RECIPE

Custom made fluid hand cleanser is one of the most comfortable regular plans you can make. It indeed doesn't require a formula. However, I'll give you one.

- 1/2 cup Castile cleanser fluid
- 1/2 cup refined water
- 1 T.B. nutrient E oil (discretionary)
- 1 T.B. sweet almond oil or olive oil or jojoba oil (discretionary)
- 15 drops tea tree fundamental oil
- 5-10 drops lavender fundamental oil

DIRECTIONS

In a bricklayer container or reused cleanser distributor, include the water first (to forestall bubbles) at that point the fluid Castile cleanser, trailed by the oils. Shake the fixings together.

Shake the cleanser container before utilizing, at that point squirt a limited quantity on your hands varying, flushing with water.

FORMULA NOTES

You don't need to utilize the fundamental oils I add to my cleanser. You're free to avoid the essential oils or investigation with different choices. In case you're using this cleanser with little youngsters, I prescribe skirting the fundamental peppermint oil, just to be wary.

The oil and nutrient E added to saturate the skin. You're free to avoid these on the off chance that you'd like. The oil won't mix with the water, so you'll have to shake the cleanser before use delicately.

Castile cleanser is a concentrated characteristic vegetable-based "cleanser" that significantly varies from the harmful detergents we are familiar with on store racks.

when you bring water into an item, you generally risk presenting microscopic organisms, so use water-based items rapidly.

CHAPTER 3
WHEN TO USE HAND SANITIZER

THE MOST EFFECTIVE METHOD TO UTILIZE HAND SANITIZER

Significantly, you use hand sanitizer appropriately to guarantee it carries out the responsibility it's intended to do – dispose of germs before they can spread:

Try not to Use Hand Sanitizer if Your Hands are Dirty: Hand sanitizers not designed to clean your hands. They intended to sterilize Residue like oil or soil will forestall hand sanitizers from entering down to your skin.

Utilize the Right Amount: When it comes to hand sanitizer, less doesn't mean more. You have to apply enough to cover all aspects of your hands thoroughly. Remember about the rear of them or your fingers!

Focus on It Until Your Hands Are Dry: This way; you can be sure that it's come into contact with all the most significant surfaces.

At the point when joined with other precaution measures (like legitimate handwashing and exhaustive touch-point cleaning), utilizing hand sanitizer will assist with keeping you (and everybody in your structure!) ensured against influenza and different ailments.

Step by step instructions to make your hand sanitizer: What you have to know

A hand sanitizer is your best protection against infections when you're out getting things done and can't find a workable pace to wash your hands. As per the CDC, the ideal approach to remain secure is to wash your hands for 20 seconds after coming back from an open spot. When in doubt, you ought to abstain from contacting your nose, eyes, or mouth with unwashed hands.

If you're as of now utilizing a hand sanitizer, ensure it has in any event 60% liquor. Some hand sanitizers are sans alcohol, and these won't be as powerful in eliminating microorganisms and infections. The right method for utilizing a hand sanitizer is to apply it generously to your hands and rub them together until the gel bubbles. Interest for hand sanitizers has shot through the rooftop in the wake of the coronavirus, and in case you're coming up short, you can undoubtedly make some at home.

Two things to know about when utilizing hand sanitizer is that you have to rub it into your hand until your hands are dry. What's more, if your hands are oily or filthy, you should wash them first with cleanser and water.

In light, here are a few hints for utilizing hand sanitizer successfully.

Splash or apply the sanitizer to the palm of one hand.

Altogether rub your hands together. Ensure you spread the whole surface of your hands and every one of your fingers.

Keep scouring for 30 to 60 seconds or until your hands are dry. It can take at any rate 60 seconds, and in some cases longer, for hand sanitizer to kill most germs.

WHY IS PROPER CLEANING NECESSARY FOR HANDS?

Appropriately cleaning your hands is perhaps the most ideal approaches to stop the spread of germs and infections, and to guarantee you don't become ill yourself. As it may, if you don't approach cleanser and clean water, or in case you're all over the place and not even close to a sink, you should convey hand sanitizer to secure your wellbeing.

Just like no uncertainty mindful, jugs of hand sanitizer (Purell, Wet Ones, and such) sell out rapidly during general wellbeing emergencies. Be that as it may, don't stress—making your hand sanitizer is amazingly simple. You simply must be cautious you don't destroy it.

Ensure that the devices you use for blending are appropriately purified; else you could defile the entire thing. Additionally, the World Health Organization prescribes, letting your mixture sit for at least 72 hours after you're finished. That way, the sanitizer has the opportunity to slaughter any microscopic organisms that may have presented during the blending procedure.

(Note: To repeat, nothing beats washing your hands. Hand sanitizer—even the good, expertly made stuff—ought to consistently be a final hotel.)

We have two plans for you, and connections to discover the fixings. The first is one you can stuff you likely as of now have in your cupboards and under the sink, so it's successful in crisis circumstances. The following formula is progressively mind-boggling, however simple to make on the off chance that you have the opportunity to do shopping and preparing of time.

Germs are all over the place! They can get onto hands and things we contact during the day by day exercises and make you debilitated. Cleaning hands at essential occasions with cleanser and water or hand sanitizer is one of the most significant advances you can take to stay away from becoming ill and spreading germs to everyone around you.

CHAPTER 4
HAND WASHING WITH SANITIZER AND WATER

There are significant contrasts between washing hands with cleanser and water furthermore, cleaning them with hand sanitizer. For instance, liquor based hand sanitizers don't execute ALL kinds of germs, for example, a stomach bug called norovirus, a few parasites, and Clostridium difficile, which causes severe looseness of the bowels. Hand sanitizers likewise may not expel poisonous synthetic substances, for example, pesticides and substantial metals like lead. Handwashing decreases the measures of a wide range of germs, pesticides, and minerals on hands. They realized when to clean your hands and which technique to utilize will give you the most obvious opportunity with regards to forestalling ailment.

WOULD IT BE GOOD FOR ME TO USE HAND SANITIZER?

Suitably cleaning your hands is maybe the best ways to deal with stop the spread of germs and contaminations, and to promise you won't turn out to be sick yourself. Nevertheless, if you don't move toward chemical and clean water, or on the off chance that you're everywhere and off by a long shot to a sink, you ought to pass close by sanitizer to make sure about your prosperity.

Much the same as no vulnerability careful, containers of hand sanitizer (Purell, Wet Ones, and such) sell out quickly during general prosperity crises. In any case, don't pressure—making your hand sanitizer is incredibly straightforward. You necessarily should be careful you don't devastate it. Guarantee that the gadgets you use for mixing are suitably filtered; else you could pollute the whole thing. Moreover, the World Health Organization recommends letting your blend sit for in any event 72 hours after done. That way, the sanitizer has the chance to butcher any minute life forms that may have introduced during the mixing system.

(Note: To rehash, nothing beats washing your hands. Hand sanitizer—even the authentic, expertly made stuff—should reliably be the last lodging.)

WHAT TYPE OF HAND SANITIZER SHOULD YOU USE?

1. We genuinely have two designs for you, and associations with find the fixings. The first you can make with stuff you starting at now have in your pantries and under the sink, so it's useful in emergency conditions. The ensuing equation is logically excellent, anyway easy to make case you get the opportunity to do some shopping and getting ready of time.
2. Utilize a hand sanitizer that contains at any rate 60% liquor.
3. Regulate little youngsters when they use hand sanitizer to forestall gulping liquor, particularly in schools and childcare offices.

HOW TO USE HAND SANITIZER?

1. Apply. Put enough item on hands to spread all surfaces.
2. Rub hands together, until hands feel dry.
3. It should take around 20 seconds.
4. Note: Do not wash or wipe off the hand
5. Sanitizer before it's dry; it may not also work against germs.

WHEN DOES HAND SANITIZER DOES NOT WORK?

Hand sanitizers may not be as successful when hands are unmistakably messy or oily.

Why? Numerous investigations show that hand sanitizers function admirably in clinical settings like emergency clinics, where hands come into contact with germs yet by, and large are not vigorously filthy or oily 16. A few information likewise show that hand sanitizers may function admirably against specific sorts of germs on marginally dirty hands 17,18. Be that as it may, hands may turn out to be exceptionally oily or dirtied in network settings, for example, after individuals handle nourishment, play sports, work in the nursery, or go outdoors or angling. At the point when hands are vigorously grimy or oily, hand sanitizers may not function admirably. Hand washing with cleanser and water suggested in such conditions.

Hand sanitizers probably won't evacuate destructive synthetic compounds, similar to pesticides and substantial metals, from hands.

Why? Albeit hardly any examinations have led, hand sanitizers most likely can't evacuate or inactivate numerous kinds of destructive synthetic concoctions. In one study, individuals who revealed utilizing hand sanitizer to clean hands had expanded degrees of pesticides in their bodies 19. If hands have contacted unsafe synthetic substances, wash cautiously with cleanser and water (or as coordinated by a toxic substance control focus).

If water are not accessible, utilize a hand sanitizer that contains at any rate 60% liquor.

Why? Numerous investigations have discovered that sanitizers with a liquor fixation between 60–95% are more compelling at eliminating germs than those with a lower liquor focus or non-liquor based hand sanitizers 16,20. Hand sanitizers without 60-95% liquor 1) may not work similarly well for some kinds of germs, and 2) just lessen the development of bacteria as opposed to murder them out and out.

When utilizing hand sanitizer, apply the item to the palm of one hand (read the mark to gain proficiency with the right sum) and rub the piece everywhere throughout the surfaces of your hands until your hands are dry.

Why? The means for hand sanitizer use depend on a streamlined technique prescribed by CDC 21. Teaching individuals to cover all surfaces of two hands with hand sanitizer has been found to give comparative sanitization adequacy as giving itemized steps to focusing available sanitizer 22.

Gulping liquor based hand sanitizers can cause liquor harming.

Why? Ethyl liquor (ethanol)- based hand sanitizers sheltered when utilized as coordinated, 23 however they can cause liquor harming if individual swallows over a few pieces

From 2011 – 2015, focuses got almost 85,000 calls about hand sanitizer exposures among kids 25. Kids might probably swallow hand sanitizers that are scented, splendidly shaded, or alluringly bundled. Hand sanitizers ought to be put away out of the span of little youngsters and ought to utilize with grown-up supervision. Kid-safe tops could likewise help lessen hand sanitizer-related poisonings among small kids 24. More established kids and grown-ups may intentionally swallow hand sanitizers to get alcoholic

CHAPTER 5
WHERE DO BACTERIAL INFECTIONS GENERATE

DECREASED SUSCEPTIBILITY OF BACTERIA TO CLEANING AGENTS

The decreased weakness of microscopic organisms to sterile specialists can either be an inborn trait of animal types or can be an Gained quality. A few reports have depicted strains of microscopic organisms that seem to have procured diminished vulnerability (at the point when characterized by MICs built up in vitro) to specific sterilizers (e.g., chlorhexidine, quaternary ammonium mixes, and triclosan). Nonetheless, because of the disinfectant focuses that are utilized by HCWs are regularly significantly higher than the MICs of strains with diminished clean defenselessness, the clinical significance of the In-vitro discoveries is sketchy—for instance, certain strains. Of MRSA have chlorhexidine and quaternary ammonium compound MICs that are a few overlaps higher than methicillin-susceptible strains and certain strains of S. aureus have Raised MICs to triclosan. In any case, such strains.

Were promptly restrained by the convergences of these germ-killers that utilized by rehearsing HCWs. The depiction of a triclosan-safe bacterial chemical has raised the subject of whether protection from this operator may create

More promptly than to other disinfectant specialists. Furthermore, uncovering Pseudomonas strains containing the MexABOprM efflux framework to triclosan may choose for freaks that are impervious to different anti-microbials, including fluoroquinolones. Further examinations expected to decide if diminished helplessness to disinfectant operators is of epidemiologic importance and whether protection from germicides has any Effect on the commonness of anti-infection safe strains

All through some random workday, representatives go through their hands to compose a report, warmly greet another customer, open entryways and considerably more. These exercises open hands to harmful germs and microbes. The ailment is connected to efficiency misfortune, costing businesses $225.8 billion yearly in the U.S. Taking into account that hands transmit 80 per cent of all diseases, it's essential to actualize a viable hand cleanliness program busy working.

Americans invest more energy Monday through Friday at the work environment than anyplace else, including their home. Furthermore, 90 per cent of office labourers will come to work in any event, when they are wiped out, to some degree because of an ever-developing workload. It makes the working environment a hotbed for germs and microorganisms. Consistently, this season's cold virus costs organizations $10.4 billion in direct expenses for hospitalizations and outpatient visits for grown-ups, as indicated by the CDC. What's more, the current year's influenza season could be awful than ordinary as specialists notice that the current year's influenza antibody may just be 10 per cent effective.

The uplifting news? Legitimate hand cleanliness consistence can lessen truancy and related expenses by 40 per cent. While washing hands with cleanser and water are the ideal approach to guarantee hands appropriately cleaned and freed of germs, and it isn't always a suitable alternative. Nonetheless, there is a straightforward arrangement: hand sanitizer. the (WHO), hand sanitizer probably the best instrument accessible to abstain from becoming ill. By setting hand sanitizer in key areas all through the workplace, and other high traffic zones, you can urge representatives to improve their hand cleanliness and make the workplace a more beneficial workspace.

CRITICAL LOCATIONS FOR HAND SANITIZER

Associations that empower the average utilization of hand sanitizer will, in general, have more advantageous labourers. An examination included in BMC Infectious Diseases found that office laboured to utilize a liquor based hand sanitizer, at any rate, multiple times every workday were around 66% more averse to become ill than the individuals who proceeded to wash their hands simply.

A 2015 study found that while 92 per cent of Americans trust it's essential to wash their hands in the wake of utilizing an open bathroom, just 66 per cent of them follow through. Over 33% of review respondents confessed to skipping cleanser and flushing with water. It was extra critical to give hand sanitizer in the bathroom. That worker is in a surge and doesn't think to stop and wash with cleanser and water, providing cement sinks, and at the entryways guarantees, germs don't get away from the bathroom.

The ideal approach to remind representatives to utilize hand sanitizer is by making it effectively open and consistently inside sight. It's critical to put hand sanitizer close and around high-contact surfaces and familiarity, including:

Passageways and ways out. A single handle might be the reason for a broad ailment in the work environment. Truth be told, new research demonstrated that an inside two to four hours, an infection set on a door handle was gotten by 40 to 60 per cent of labourers and guests inside the facility. Notwithstanding much of the time sterilizing door handles, light switches and other high-contact surfaces inside the work environment, try to likewise give a hand disinfecting station close by to confine the spread of disease.

Cafeterias, nourishment courts and break rooms, and if nourishment is overcome with germ-ridden hands, it's anything but difficult to process the germs and become tainted with a few maladies. Probably the germiest hotspot in an office is the lounge and kitchen, as per an NSF International study. In spite of the fact that hand sanitizer isn't a trade for any individual who gets ready nourishment, it can help take out specific germs.

Meeting rooms. Meeting rooms are frequently pressed with workers, customers and different guests who trade handshakes, subsequently swapping germs. By furnishing visitors and representatives with a simple to-get to hand disinfecting station, either close to the entryway or at the table permits them to protect their hands against germs when the gathering happens.

Representative work areas. Work areas, telephones, P.C. consoles and P.C. mice are key germ move focuses on the grounds that individuals contact them so frequently. Taking into account that workers spend most of their day at their work areas where they additionally eat, drink and even hack and wheeze, work areas become "a minefield of infections" which can live for up to three days. Putting singular hand sanitizers at work areas keeps hand cleanliness close enough.

High traffic territories. Giving hand sanitizer outside of the workplace is likewise significant. High-traffic zones like air terminal terminals, shopping centre lobbies and recreational focuses should offer hand cleanliness stations to guarantee guests remain as sound as could be expected under the circumstances. In addition to the fact that this keeps high-traffic territories clean, it improves the picture of the air terminal, shopping centre or rec focus.

EXCHANGE COUNTERS

In a recent report, specialists swabbed $1 greenbacks from a bank and found many types of microorganisms living on them. Extra research has discovered pathogens, for example, E. coli, salmonella and staphylococcus aureus on paper cash, which all could prompt genuine illness. In the wake of dealing with money, it's critical to clean your hands, particularly in case you're going to expend nourishment presently subsequently. Keeping hand sanitizer close to exchange territories, for example, the cafeteria registration counter reminds individuals to take part close by cleanliness when it's required most.

CHOOSING THE RIGHT-HAND SANITIZER

While giving hand sanitizer at key areas all through the work environment is basic to battling representative sickness and non-attendance, it works best to give the correct sort of sanitizer. Make a point to utilize a liquor based hand sanitizer that contains in any event 70 per cent liquor. The higher liquor rate will typically convert into higher adequacy. Search for items with a 5-log least kill rate (99.999%) – which are multiple times more powerful than 3-log (99.9%) sanitizers.

Consider utilizing froth hand sanitizers, as 84 per cent of grown-ups lean toward froth sanitizer over clingy gel. It's likewise best to utilize sanitizers that contain creams to forestall skin dryness, and are scent and colour allowed to decrease potential hypersensitive responses and skin aggravations.

EMPOWERING HAND HYGIENE

A total hand cleanliness program goes past, giving the correct items. While having divider mounted hand sterilizing distributors and jugs on surfaces in and approach germ hotspots are fundamental to improving the soundness of your labourers, it's just advantageous if labourers consistently use them.

Give banners, flyers, inside pamphlets and data loads up close to gadgets with suggestions to clean hands and offer brisk, simple realities about hand cleanliness. These materials ought to likewise remember data for how to appropriately utilize and apply hand sanitizer as indicated by the 6 Step Method prescribed by the World Health Organization, to guarantee the right sum is utilized and spread to cover all surfaces of two hands. Also, businesses should offer instructive workshops and gatherings during the time to educate and remind representatives on how they can improve their wellbeing with hand cleanliness best practices.

As a business, it's critical to lead change with a model. Urge labourers to utilize sanitizer regularly by doing so yourself. Remember to load up available cleanliness tops off during the cold and influenza season too. In conclusion, it's imperative to remind labourers to take a day off when essential so as to get germs far from the workplace and other solid specialists.

STERILIZING THE WORKPLACE

Utilizing hand sanitizer lessens microbial checks and executes numerous unsafe germs that could taint labourers with this season's flu virus and different infections. So as to keep the work environment a sound and flourishing condition, it's important that businesses consider the strength of their representatives. Giving hand sanitizer to workers, at work areas and in shared regions, is similarly as fundamental as giving the correct gear and devices to carry out their responsibility.

CHAPTER 6
CONCLUSION

Hand sanitizer is convenient in a hurried approach to help forestall the spread of germs when cleanser and water aren't accessible. Liquor based hand sanitizers can help keep you safe and decrease the spread of the novel coronavirus.

If you are making some hard memories discovering hand sanitizer at your nearby stores, you can find a way to make your own. You just need a couple of fixings, for example, scouring liquor, aloe vera gel, and an essential oil or lemon juice.

Even though hand sanitizers can be a viable method for disposing of germs, wellbeing specialists despite everything prescribe hand washing at whatever point conceivable to keep your hands liberated from infection-causing infections and different bacteria.

As indicated by my exploration, the best and most straightforward approach to remain solid is to wash your hands. This reality made me need to realize what is progressively viable for eliminating germs on your hands at school - cleanser or hand sanitizer? I guessed that if you use sanitizer or cleanser to clean your hands at school, at that point utilizing sanitizer will evacuate the most germs since utilizing sanitizer doesn't expect you to contact the sink spigot. The underlying example I took from the sink fixture, knapsack and iPad all developed viruses, so this demonstrated we do get germs on our hands in the wake of contacting these articles. My control dish didn't establish any infections, and this reflects my Petri dishes were perfect and not sullied toward the beginning of my trial. The information indicated that washing hands with cleanser and water successfully decreased the number of germs on hands by 12-half. Utilizing hand sanitizer to clean hands diminished the amount of bacteria present by 35-70%. The consequences of my investigation, Soap versus Sanitizer, demonstrated my theory is right since hand sanitizer is typical of 146% more viable than cleanser at cleaning our hands at school. This data picked up from my trial is significant because it tends to utilized to help stop the germs at school and keep understudies and educators reliable. I can prescribe that understudies ought to be permitted to use sanitizer as opposed to washing their hands with cleanser, or that the school should introduce programmed touchless fixtures in the restrooms. The examination could extend by taking various examples from each surface or by testing objects in different areas outside of the school. Testing should be possible on the viability of cleanser and sanitizer on noticeably filthy hands, or the adequacy of various kinds of shampoos or a wide range of hand sanitizers.

www.ingramcontent.com/pod-product-compliance
Lightning Source LLC
Chambersburg PA
CBHW050326220526
45465CB00005B/2151